THE OBESITY CODE

Health Dangers Related With Obesity, Treatments, Guide On Successful Weight loss Programs With Foods & Recipes

Jason Fu-chi

INTRODUCTION

Obesity isn't just a restorative idea. It is a relentless restorative contamination that can provoke diabetes, hypertension, Obesity related cardiovascular ailment, for instance, coronary ailment, gallstones, and other consistent illnesses.

Obesity is a danger factor for different sicknesses.

Obesity is difficult to treat and has a high lose the faith rate. A large number individuals who shed pounds recover the weight inside five years.

Regardless of the way that remedies and diets can help, the treatment of Obesity can't be a present minute "fix" anyway should be an enduring duty to proper eating routine affinities, extended physical activity, and normal exercise.

The goal of treatment should be to achieve and keep up a "progressively valuable weight," not so much an ideal weight.

A key bit of transforming into a Healthier you is choosing strong choices. This bit of the book will give you a segment of the gadgets to stay on track. One of the least perplexing and best cool headed choices you can make is to fathom what you are eating. Cooking at home is one sure fire way to deal with plan and screen calories, parcel sizes, supplements, and the sum of that other incredible stuff.

WHAT IS OBESITY

The importance of obesity varies depending upon what one examines. At the point when all is said in done, overweight and obesity show a weight more unmistakable than what is sound. obesity is a steady condition portrayed by an excess proportion of muscle versus fat.

 A particular proportion of muscle versus fat is fundamental for taking care of imperativeness, heat assurance, shock maintenance, and various limits.

Weight file best describes huskiness. A person's height and weight chooses their weight file. The weight record (BMI) moves toward a person's heap in kilograms (kg) disconnected by their height in meters (m) squared (more information will be found later in the article). Since BMI depicts body weight relative with stature, there is a strong association with hard and fast muscle to fat proportion content in adults. An adult who has a BMI of 25-29.9 is overweight, and an adult who has a BMI more than 30 is huge. A person with a BMI of 18.5-24.9 has a standard weight. An individual is unreasonably fat (ludicrous chubbiness) if their BMI is more than 40.

HEALTH DANGERS RELATED WITH OBESITY

Obesity isn't just a restorative idea; it is destructive to one's prosperity as it is a danger factor for certain conditions. In the United States, roughly 112,000 passings for every year are direct related to rotundity, and most of these passings are in patients with a BMI more than 30. Patients with a BMI more than 40 have a reduced future. Obesity furthermore assembles the threat of working up different consistent disorders, including the going with:

- **Insulin Obstruction:** Insulin is significant for the vehicle of blood glucose (sugar) into the cells of muscle and fat (which the body uses for essentialness). By moving glucose into cells, insulin keeps the blood glucose levels in the run of the mill go. Insulin hindrance (IR) is the condition whereby there is diminished reasonability of insulin in delivery glucose (sugar) into cells. Fat cells are more insulin safe than muscle cells; henceforth, one huge purpose behind insulin resistance is robustness. The pancreas from the start responds to insulin deterrent by making more insulin. For whatever period of time that the pancreas can convey enough insulin to overcome this resistance, blood glucose levels remain normal. This insulin resistance state (portrayed by run of the mill blood glucose levels and high insulin levels) can prop up for a significant long time. At the point when the pancreas can never again remain mindful of conveying huge degrees of insulin, blood glucose levels begin to rise, achieving type 2 diabetes, thusly insulin resistance is a pre-diabetes condition.

- **Type 2 (grown-up starting) diabetes:** The risk of type 2 diabetes increases with the degree and length of heftiness. Type 2 diabetes is connected with central huskiness; a person with central weight has wealth fat around his/her waist.

- **(Hypertension):** Hypertension is fundamental among robust adults. A Norwegian report showed that weight expansion would all in all addition beat in women more on a very basic level than in men.

- Elevated cholesterol (hypercholesterolemia)

- Stroke (cerebrovascular disaster or CVA)

- **Cancer:** heftiness is a peril factor for Cancer of the colon in individuals, infection of the rectum and prostate in men, and danger of the gallbladder and uterus in women. Strength may in like manner be connected with chest infection, particularly in postmenopausal women. Fat tissue is critical in the age of estrogen, and postponed prologue to raised degrees of estrogen constructs the risk of chest ailment.

- Gallstones

- Gout and gouty joint torment

- Osteoarthritis: (degenerative joint torment) of the knees, hips, and the lower back

- Rest apnea

MOST NORMAL REASONS FOR OBESITY

The amicability between calorie confirmation and imperativeness utilization chooses a person's weight. If an individual eats a bigger number of calories than the individual expends (uses), the individual puts on weight (the body will store the excess imperativeness as fat). In case an individual eats less calories than the individual uses, the individual will get more slender. Thusly, the most generally perceived purposes behind weight are pigging out and physical inactivity. Finally, body weight is the eventual outcome of innate characteristics, assimilation, condition, direct, and culture.

Physical latency: Stationary people devour less calories than people who are dynamic. The National Health and Nutrition Examination Survey (NHANES) showed a strong connections between's physical inertness and weight gain in the two sexual orientations.

Indulging: Gorging prompts weight gain, especially if the eating routine is high in fat. Sustenances high in fat or sugar (for example, cheap nourishment, scorched sustenance, and pastries) have high essentialness thickness (nourishment sources that have a lot of calories in an unassuming amount of sustenance).

Epidemiologic examinations have demonstrated that diets high in fat add to weight gain.

Innate characteristics: An individual will undoubtedly make heftiness if one or the two gatekeepers are fat. Inherited characteristics also impact hormones related with fat rule. For example, one genetic purpose behind corpulence is leptin insufficiency. Leptin is a hormone made in fat cells and in the placenta. Leptin controls weight by hailing the cerebrum to eat less when muscle versus fat stores are unreasonably high. In case, for no good reason, the body can't make enough leptin or leptin can't hail the cerebrum to eat less, this control is lost, and weight occurs. The activity of leptin swap as a treatment for obesity is under scrutiny.

WHAT ARE OTHER FACTORS ASSOCIATED WITH OBESITY

Ethnicity: Ethnicity segments may affect the hour of starting and the speed of weight gain. African-American women and Hispanic women will when all is said in done experience weight increment earlier in life than Caucasians and Asians, and age-adjusted chubbiness rates are higher in these social occasions. Non-Hispanic dull men and Hispanic men have a higher chunkiness rate then non-Hispanic white men, yet the differentiation in inescapability is in a general sense not actually in women.

Youth weight: A person's heap during immaturity, the secondary school years, and early adulthood may in like manner sway the improvement of adult weight. In this way, lessening the transcendence of youth obesity is one of the regions to focus on in the fight against huskiness. For example,

Being to some degree overweight in the mid 20s was associated with a huge pace of forcefulness by age 35;

Being overweight during progressively settled pre-adulthood is significantly farsighted of adult weight, especially if a parent is furthermore stoutness;

Being overweight during the secondary school years is even a progressively unmistakable pointer of adult stoutness.

METHODOLOGIES MEASURE MUSCLE VERSUS FAT

BMI is a decided worth and approximates the muscle to fat ratio's. Everything considered evaluating a person's muscle versus fat proportion isn't basic and is as often as possible wrong without mindful checking of the techniques. The going with techniques require remarkable rigging, arranged personnel, can be over the top, and some are only open in certain investigation workplaces.

Submerged checking (hydrostatic measuring): This methodology checks an individual submerged and subsequently determines fit weight (muscle) and muscle to fat proportion. This technique is one of the most definite ones; in any case, the equipment is costly.

Body POD: The BOD POD is an automated, egg-shaped chamber. Using a comparable whole body estimation rule as hydrostatic measuring, the BOD POD gauges a subject's mass and volume, from which their whole body thickness is settled.

Using this data, muscle versus fat and fit mass would then have the option to be resolved.

Skin calipers: This system gauges the skinfold thickness of the layer of fat essentially under the skin in a couple of bits of the body with calipers (a metal instrument like forceps); the results are then used to calculate the degree of muscle versus fat.

Bioelectric impedance examination (BIA): There are two methods for the BIA. One remembers staying for a remarkable scale with footpads.

A harmless proportion of electrical stream is sent through the body, and a while later degree of muscle versus fat is resolved. The other sort of BIA incorporates cathodes that are normally put on a wrist and a lower leg and on the rear of the right hand and on the most elevated purpose of the foot. The alteration in voltage between the anodes is evaluated. The person's muscle to fat proportion is then decided from the delayed consequences of the BIA. Directly off the bat, this system showed variable results. More forward-thinking equipment and systems for assessment seem to have improved this technique.

WHAT IS THE WEIGHT RECORD (BMI)

The weight record (BMI) is a now the estimation of choice for certain specialists and examiners thinking about Obesity.

The BMI uses a numerical formula that records for both a person's weight and stature.

The BMI estimation, in any case, speaks to a segment of undefined issues from the weight-for-stature tables. Only one out of every odd individual agrees on the cutoff centers for "strong" versus "unwanted" BMI ranges. BMI also doesn't give information on a person's degree of muscle to fat proportion. Regardless, like the weight-for-stature table, BMI is a useful general principle and is a nice estimator of muscle versus fat for most adults 19 and 70 years of age. In any case, it may not be a definite estimation of muscle versus fat for weight lifters, certain contenders, and pregnant women.

The BMI ascends to a person's heap in kilograms segregated by stature in meters squared (BMI = kg/m2). To process the BMI using pounds, parcel the weight in pounds by the stature in inches squared and copy the result by 703.

It is basic to understand what "sound weight" means. Sound weight is portrayed as a weight record (BMI) equal to or more noticeable than 19 and under 25 among all people 20 years of age or over. Generally, huskiness is portrayed as a weight document (BMI) proportionate to or more critical than 30, which approximates 30 pounds of excess weight.

The World Health Organization uses a gathering system using the BMI to describe overweight and weight.

A BMI of 25 to 29.9 is described as a "pre-heavy."

A BMI of 30 to 34.99 is described as "heavy class I."

A BMI of 35 to 39.99 is described as "heavy class II."

A BMI of or more unmistakable than 40.00 is described as "forceful class III."

Does it have any kind of effect where muscle to fat proportion is found? (Is it progressively awful to be an "apple" or a "pear"?)

Concern is composed not exactly at how much fat an individual has yet what's more where that fat is arranged on the body. The case of muscle to fat proportion allocation will when all is said in done difference in individuals.

When in doubt, women accumulate fat in their hips and

rump, giving their figures a "pear" shape. Men, of course, commonly assemble fat around the waist, giving them a more noteworthy measure of an "apple" shape. (This is authentically not a firm principle; a couple of men are pear-shaped and a couple of women become apple-framed, particularly after menopause.)

Apple-formed people whose fat is amassed by and large in the stomach will undoubtedly make a significant part of the restorative issues related with weight. They are at extended prosperity peril because of their fat spread. While chubbiness of any kind is a prosperity peril, it is more brilliant to be a pear than an apple.

In order to sort the sorts of normal item, pros have developed an essential strategy to choose in the event that someone is an apple or a pear. The estimation is called belly to-hip extent. To find a person's guts to-hip extent measure the waist at its most secure point, and a while later measure the hips at the most loosened up point;

separate the waist estimation by the hip estimation. For example, a woman with a 35-inch waist and 46-inch hips would have a guts to-hip extent of 0.76 (35 secluded by 46 = 0.76).

Women with waist to-hip extents of more than 0.8 and men with guts to-hip extents of more than 1.0 are "apples."

Another horrendous technique for assessing the proportion of a person's stomach fat is by evaluating the belly border. Men with a midsection blueprint of 40 inches or progressively essential and women with a belly circuit of 35 inches or increasingly noticeable are considered to have extended prosperity risks related to weight.

WHAT SHOULD BE POSSIBLE ABOUT WEIGHT

Regularly, obesity prompts a strenuous eating routine with desires for going to the "flawless body weight." Some proportion of weight decrease may be developed, anyway the shed pounds normally quickly returns. A large number individuals who get progressively fit recoup the weight inside five years. Undeniably a dynamically incredible, strong treatment for heaviness must be found.

We need to get comfortable with the explanations behind bulkiness, and a short time later we need to change the habits in which we treat it. Right when heaviness is recognized as an unending disease, it will be managed like other relentless ailments, for instance, diabetes and hypertension. The treatment of huskiness can't be a present minute "fix" anyway should be a consistent profound established methodology.

Obesity treatment must perceive that in any event, unassuming weight decrease can be profitable. For example, an inconspicuous weight decrease of 5%-10% of the basic weight, and long stretch upkeep of that weight decrease can bring critical prosperity gains, including Cut down heartbeat;

Diminished blood levels of cholesterol; Diminished threat of type 2 (grown-up starting) diabetes (In the Nurses Health

Study, women who lost 5 kilograms [11 pounds] of weight decreased their risk of diabetes significantly or more.);

Decreased plausibility of stroke;

Decreased challenges of coronary disease;

Decreased all around mortality.

It isn't essential to achieve a "flawless weight" to get therapeutic favorable circumstances from heaviness treatment. Or maybe, the target of treatment should be to reach and hold to an "increasingly gainful weight." The emphasis of treatment should be to concentrate on the system of profound established strong living, including eating even more commendably and extending physical activity.

Altogether, the target in overseeing obesity is to achieve and keep up an "increasingly worthwhile weight."

THE JOB OF PHYSICAL ACTIVITIES AND EXERCISE IN WEIGHT

The National Health and Examination Survey (NHANES I) demonstrated that people who make part in limited recreational move will undoubtedly put on weight than continuously unique people. Various examinations have exhibited that people who take an interest in common strenuous activity put on less weight than stationary people.

Physical development and exercise help expend calories. The proportion of calories devoured depends upon the sort, length, and intensity of the development. It in like manner depends upon the weight of the person. A 200-pound individual will expend a more noteworthy number of calories running 1 mile than a 120-pound individual, in light of the fact that made by passing on those extra 80 pounds must be figured in. In any case, practice as a treatment for weight is best when gotten together with an eating routine and get-solid arrangement. Exercise alone without dietary changes will limitedly influence weight since one needs to rehearse a lot to simply lose 1 pound. In any case standard exercise is a noteworthy bit of a strong lifestyle to keep up a sound load to the extent that this would be possible. Another favored situation of standard practice as a significant part of a get-solid arrangement is a progressively conspicuous loss of muscle to fat proportion versus fit muscle appeared differently in relation to the people who diet alone.

EXERCISE PRECAUTIONARY MEASURES

The going with people should direct a master before overpowering movement:

- Men over age 40 or women over age 50

- People with heart or lung disorder, asthma, joint torment, or osteoporosis People who experience chest weight or anguish with exertion, or who make depletion or curtness of breath viably

- People with conditions or lifestyle factors that development their threat of making coronary sickness, for instance, hypertension, diabetes, cigarette smoking, high blood cholesterol, or having family members with early starting cardiovascular disappointments and coronary disease

- A understanding who is fat.

WHAT IS THE JOB OF DIET IN THE TREATMENT OF OBESITY

The essential target of devouring less calories is to stop further weight gain. The accompanying target is to develop commonsense weight decrease destinations. While the ideal weight looks at to a BMI of 20-25, this is difficult to achieve for certain people. Thusly, accomplishment is higher when a goal is set to lose 10%-15% of benchmark weight as opposed to 20%-30% or progressively unmistakable. It is similarly basic to review that any weight decline in a hefty individual would realize restorative focal points.

One incredible way to deal with get progressively fit is to eat less calories. One pound is comparable to 3,500 calories. Toward the day's end, you have to expend 3,500 a more prominent number of calories than you eat up to lose 1 pound. Most adults need between 1,200-2,800 calories for every day, dependent upon body size and activity level to meet the body's imperativeness needs.

If you skirt that bowl of sweet, by then you will be one-seventh of the best way to deal with losing that pound! Losing 1 pound for consistently is a secured and reasonable way to deal with remove extra pounds. The higher the hidden heap of an individual, the more quickly he/she will achieve weight decrease. This is in light of the fact that for every 1 kilogram (2.2 pounds) of body weight, around 22 calories are required to keep up that weight. So for a woman checking 100 kilograms (220 pounds), the person being referred to would require around 2,200 calories for each day to keep up their weight, while an individual measuring 60 kilograms (132 pounds) would require just around 1,320 calories. If both ate a calorie-bound eating routine of 1,200 calories for every day, the heavier individual would get fit as a fiddle snappier. Age in like manner is a factor in calorie use. Metabolic rate will when all is said in done postponed as we age, so the more prepared an individual is, the harder it is to get increasingly fit.

General eating routine principles for achieving and (correspondingly as fundamentally) keeping up a sound weight

A secured and amazing long stretch weight decline and bolster diet needs to contain balanced, nutritious sustenances to avoid supplement deficiencies and various afflictions of absence of solid sustenance.

Eat progressively nutritious sustenances that have "low imperativeness thickness." Low essentialness thick nourishment sources contain reasonably scarcely any calories per unit weight (less calories in a great deal of sustenance). Occurrences of low imperativeness thick sustenances join vegetables, natural items, lean meat, fish, grains, and beans. For example, you can eat a gigantic volume of celery or carrots without taking in various calories.

Eat less "essentialness thick sustenances." Energy thick nourishment sources are high in fats and direct sugars. They generally have a greasy motivator in a constrained amount of sustenance. The United States government at present endorses that a strong eating routine should have under 30% fat. Fat contains double a similar number of calories per unit weight than protein or sugars. Cases of high-imperativeness thick sustenances join red meat, egg yolks, seared sustenances, high fat/sugar fast sustenances, sweets, cakes, spread, and high-fat serving of blended greens dressings. Furthermore cut down on sustenances that give calories anyway beside no sustenance, for instance, alcohol, non-diet soft drinks, and many packaged undesirable snack sustenances.

About 55% of calories in the eating routine should be from complex sugars. Eat progressively complex sugars, for instance, dim hued rice, whole grain bread, natural items, and vegetables. Keep up a key good ways from essential starches, for instance, table sugars, sweets, doughnuts, cakes, and scones. Cut down on non-diet soft drink pops, these sugary soft drinks are stacked with clear starches and calories. Clear starches cause over the top insulin release by the pancreas, and insulin progresses improvement of fat tissue.

Train yourself in examining sustenance stamps and assessing calories and serving sizes.

Insight a pro before starting any dietary changes. You pro or a nutritionist should suggest the proportion of step by step calories in your eating routine.

THE WORK OF MEDICATION IN THE TREATMENT OF OBESITY

Remedy treatment of weight should be used unmistakably in patients who have prosperity perils related to chubbiness. Drugs should be used in patients with a BMI more significant than 30 or in those with a BMI of more unmistakable than 27 who have different sicknesses, (for instance, hypertension, diabetes, high blood cholesterol) that put them in threat for making coronary ailment. Solutions should not be used for remedial reasons.

Medications should simply be used as an extra to thin down changes and a movement program.

Like eating routine and exercise, the target of medication treatment must be viable. With successful remedy treatment, one can expect a basic weight decrease of at any rate 5 pounds during the important month of treatment, and a total weight decrease of 10%-15% of the basic body weight. It is also basic to review that these solutions conceivably work when they are taken. Exactly when they are suspended, weight gain much of the time occurs.

The first rate (class) of medication used for weight control cause reactions that duplicate the attentive tangible framework. They cause the body to feel "under tension" or "on edge." accordingly, the critical response of this class of medication is hypertension. This class of medication consolidates sibutramine (Meridia, which was evacuated the market in the U.S. in October 2010 as a result of security concerns) and phentermine (Adipex P). These prescriptions moreover decrease wanting and rustle up some fervor of totality. Hunger and finishing (satiety) are overseen by cerebrum engineered mixes called neurotransmitters. Occurrences of neural connections join serotonin, norepinephrine, and dopamine. Unfriendly to forcefulness medications that cover desiring do in that capacity by growing the level of these neurotransmitters at the crossing point (called neural association) between nerve endings in the cerebrum.

Phentermine: Phentermine (Fastin, Adipex P) - the other segment of fen/phen - covers hunger by causing an appearance of norepinephrine in the body. Phentermine alone is up 'til now available for treatment of forcefulness anyway just on a flitting premise (a large portion of a month). The fundamental responses of phentermine fuse headache, a dozing issue, trickiness, and trepidation. Fenfluramine (the fen of fen/phen) and dexfenfluramine (Redux) cover hunger generally by growing appearance of serotonin by the cells. Both fenfluramine and dexfenfluramine were pulled once again from the market in September 1997 in perspective on relationship of these two medications with pneumonic hypertension (an exceptional anyway real ailment of the stock courses in the lungs) and relationship of fen/phen with mischief to the heart valves. Since the withdrawal of fenfluramine, some have proposed joining phentermine with fluoxetine (Prozac), a mix that has been suggested as phen/ace. In any case, no clinical primers have been directed to confirm the security and sufficiency of this blend. As such, this blend isn't a recognized treatment for heftiness.

Orlistat (Xenical, alli) : The accompanying class (arrangement) of prescriptions changes the absorption of fat. Orlistat (Xenical, alli) is the primary drug of this class is U.S. FDA supported. This is a class of against weight meds called lipase inhibitors, or fat blockers. Fat from sustenance must be devoured into the body in the wake of being separated (a strategy called retention) by stomach related impetuses called lipases in the absorption tracts. By controlling the movement of lipase mixes, orlistat balances the intestinal absorption of fat by 30%. Prescriptions in this class don't impact cerebrum science. Theoretically, orlistat moreover should have inconsequential or no essential side effects (responses in various bits of the body) considering the way that the noteworthy district of action is inside the gut lumen and by no of the medicine is ingested.

The U.S. Sustenance and Drug Administration supported orlistat compartments, set apart as alli, as an over-the-counter (OTC) treatment for overweight adults in February 2007. The medicine had as of late been insisted in 1999 as an answer weight decrease help, whose brand name is Xenical. The OTC arranging has a lower estimations than arrangement Xenical.

Orlistat is recommended extraordinarily for people 18 years of age and over in mix with an eating routine and exercise schedule. People who experience issues with the digestion of sustenance or who are not overweight should not take orlistat. Overweight is portrayed by the U.S. National Institutes of Health as having a weight record (BMI) of at least 27 conspicuous.

Orlistat can be involved to multiple times every day, with each fat-containing supper. The prescription may be taken during the supper or up to one hour after the dinner. If the supper is missed or is incredibly low in fat substance, the solutions should not be taken.

The most broadly perceived manifestations of orlistat are changes in inside affinities. These fuse gas, the basic need to have a strong release, smooth poops, smooth discharge or spotting with strong releases, an extended repeat of strong releases, and the inability to control strong releases. Women may in like manner see irregularities in the menstrual cycle while taking orlistat. Responses are generally essential in the underlying scarcely any weeks consequent to beginning to take orlistat. In specific people, the responses proceed for whatever time span that they are taking the prescription.

People with diabetes, thyroid conditions, who have gotten an organ transplant, or who are taking expertly endorsed medicines that impact blood thickening should check with their primary care physician before using OTC orlistat (alli), since steady participations with explicit medications are possible.

A long stretch decrease in fat ingestion can cause absence of fat-dissolvable supplements, (for instance, supplements A, D, E, K). Along these lines, patients on orlistat should get adequate supplement supplementation.

HOW CAN PEOPLE CHOOSE A SAFE AND SUCCESSFUL WEIGHT-LOSS PROGRAM?

Scientists have made tremendous strides in understanding obesity and in improving the medication treatment of this important disease. In time, better, safer, and more effective obesity medications will be available. But currently there is still no "magic cure" for obesity. The best and safest way to lose fat and keep it off is through a commitment to a lifelong process of proper diet and regular exercise.

Medications should be

considered helpful adjuncts to diet and exercise for patients whose health risk from obesity clearly outweigh the potential side effects of the medications. Medications should be prescribed by doctors familiar with the patients' conditions and with the use of the medications. Medication(s) and other "herbal" preparations with unproven effectiveness and safety should be avoided.

Almost any of the commercial weight-loss programs can work but only if they motivate you sufficiently to decrease the amount of calories you eat or increase the amount of calories you burn each day (or both). What elements of a weight-loss program should a consumer look for in judging its potential for safe and successful weight loss? A responsible and safe weight-loss program should be able to document for you the five following features:

The diet should be safe. It should include all of the recommended daily allowances (RDAs) for vitamins, minerals, and protein. The weight-loss diet should be low in calories (energy) only, not in essential foodstuffs.

The weight-loss program should be directed toward a slow, steady weight loss unless your doctor feels your health condition would benefit from more rapid weight loss. Expect to lose only about a pound a week after the first week or two. With many calorie-restricted diets there is an initial rapid weight loss during the first one to two weeks, but this loss is largely fluid.

If you plan to lose more than 15 to 20 pounds, have any health problems, or take medication on a regular basis, you should be evaluated by your doctor before beginning your weight-loss program. A doctor can assess your general health and any medical conditions that might be affected by dieting and weight loss. Also, a physician should be able to advise you on the need for weight loss, the appropriateness of the weight-loss program, and a sensible goal of weight loss for you. If you plan to use a very low-calorie diet (a special liquid formula diet that replaces all food intake for one to four months), you should do so under the close supervision of a health care professional.

Your program should include plans for weight maintenance after the weight-loss phase is over. It is of little benefit to lose a large amount of weight only to regain it. Weight maintenance is the most difficult part of controlling weight and is not consistently implemented in weight-loss programs. The program you select should include help in permanently changing your dietary habits and level of physical activity

Researchers have made enormous walks in getting stoutness and in improving the prescription treatment of this significant infection. In time, better, more secure, and increasingly successful heftiness drugs will be accessible. Be that as it may, at present there is still no "enchantment fix" for heftiness. The best and most secure approach to lose fat and keep it off is through a pledge to a long lasting procedure of legitimate eating regimen and standard exercise. Meds ought to be viewed as accommodating extras to slim down and practice for patients whose wellbeing hazard from corpulence obviously exceed the potential reactions of the prescriptions. Meds ought to be endorsed by specialists acquainted with the patients' conditions and with the utilization of the meds. Medication(s) and other "home grown" arrangements with dubious adequacy and security ought to be kept away from.

Practically any of the business get-healthy plans can work however just on the off chance that they spur you adequately to diminish the measure of calories you eat or increment the measure of calories you consume every day (or both). What components of a get-healthy plan should a customer search for in making a decision about its potential for sheltered and effective weight reduction? A mindful and safe health improvement plan ought to have the option to record for you the five after highlights:

The eating regimen ought to be sheltered. It ought to incorporate the entirety of the prescribed every day recompenses (RDAs) for nutrients, minerals, and protein. The weight reduction diet ought to be low in calories (vitality) just, not in fundamental groceries.

The get-healthy plan ought to be coordinated toward a moderate, enduring weight reduction except if your primary care physician feels your wellbeing condition would profit by progressively fast weight reduction. Hope to lose just about a pound seven days after the primary week or two. With numerous calorie-confined eating regimens there is an underlying quick weight reduction during the first to about fourteen days, however this misfortune is to a great extent liquid.

On the off chance that you intend to lose more than 15 to 20 pounds, have any medical issues, or take medicine all the time, you ought to be assessed by your primary care physician before starting your get-healthy plan. A specialist can evaluate your general wellbeing and any ailments that may be influenced by abstaining from excessive food intake and weight reduction. Additionally, a doctor ought to have the option to prompt you on the requirement for weight reduction, the fittingness of the get-healthy plan, and a reasonable objective of weight reduction for you. On the off chance that you intend to utilize a low-calorie diet (an exceptional fluid recipe diet that replaces all nourishment admission for one to four months), you ought to do as such under the nearby supervision of a medicinal services proficient.

Your program ought to incorporate designs for weight upkeep after the weight reduction stage is finished. It is of little advantage to lose a lot of weight just to recapture it. Weight support is the most troublesome piece of controlling weight and isn't reliably executed in health improvement plans. The program you select ought to incorporate assistance in for all time changing your dietary propensities and level of physical activity.

FOODS AND RECIPES

OAT AND BUCKWHEAT MUESLI WITH PEARS AND GRAPES (DAIRY-FREE)

Eating a bowl of this super-nutritious muesli for breakfast is a heavenly method to begin a three day weekend right. The oats it contains give a lot of fiber and protein, while the pears convey iodine. Iodine is essential for the best possible working of the thyroid organ which controls the basal metabolic rate, that is, the rate at which the body devours vitality very still. Iodine lack can bring about languid thyroid action which thusly can prompt weight pick up or impede your endeavors to thin down.

Ingredients:

1/2 cups moved oats

1/2 cup puffed buckwheat

1/2 cup dried apples, cleaved

2 tsp ground cinnamon

1 cup natural pears, diced

1 cup red grapes, divided

3 tbsp dark colored sugar

Rice milk to serve

Directions:

Preheat broiler to 325°F (160°C, gas 3).

Spread oats uniformly onto a non-stick heating plate and toast in preheated broiler for around 10 minutes, blending at times. Watch oats intently when toasting as they can consume effectively.

Expel from broiler and let cool. Fill a huge earthenware or glass bowl and include water. Give drench access a cooler medium-term.

Include puffed buckwheat, dried apples, cinnamon, and dark colored sugar to splashed oats. Mix well.

Separation blend into serving bowls and top with pears and grapes. Present with rice milk.

Did you know?

Dousing improves the healthy benefit of oats as it enables catalysts to separate and kill phytic corrosive, an intensify that can obstruct the retention of numerous minerals.

WEIGHT LOSS MUFFINS

These luscious weight reduction biscuits are stuffed with fiber and protein while being very low in fat. Also, the blueberries they contain gloat an extraordinary fiber called gelatin which can restrict the measure of fat your phones retain.

Ingredients:

1 cup moved oats, absorbed 1 cup skim milk for 1-2 hours

1/2 cup unsweetened fruit purée

2 egg whites

1 cup skim milk

1 cup entire wheat flour

1/2 cup darker sugar

1 tsp heating powder

1/2 tsp heating pop

1/2 tsp salt

1 tsp cinnamon

1 cup blueberries

Directions:

Preheat broiler to 400 degrees F (200 degrees C, gas mark 6).

Beat together egg whites, oat-milk blend, and fruit purée. Join dry fixings in a different bowl.

Add fluid fixings to dry fixings and blend until simply joined (don't over-blend). Overlap in blueberries.

Fill 12 paper biscuit cups with player (around 66% full). Heat for 20 minutes or until done.

LOW GLYCEMIC RASPBERRY MUFFINS

This biscuit formula is an unquestionable requirement pursue the individuals who love biscuits however are worried about the high measure of basic sugars in many biscuits. This formula utilizes low-glycemic biscuit fixings, including raspberries, soy flour, and entire wheat flour. It likewise includes cinnamon which assists bring down the glycemic list of these flavorful weight reduction biscuits.

Ingredients:

1/2 cups entire wheat flour

1/2 cup soy flour

2 tsp preparing powder

1/3 cup dark colored sugar

2 tsp cinnamon

2 egg whites

1 cup soy milk

2 Tbsp canola oil

1 cup raspberries

Directions:

Preheat stove to 375°F (190°C, gas mark 5).

Consolidate dry fixings in a huge bowl. Whisk together egg whites, soy milk, and canola oil in a different bowl.

Add wet fixings to dry fixings and blend until simply mixed (don't over-blend). Crease in raspberries.

Fill 12 paper biscuit cups with hitter (around 66% full). Prepare until an analyzer toothpick confesses all, around 15-20 minutes.

LEEK AND GARLIC OMELET

The primary fixing in this weight reduction formula is egg whites, which are at the highest point of wellness models and famous people's arrangements of most loved weight reduction nourishments as they are amazing wellspring of dietary protein however low in calories and fat. Likewise garlic is normally used to avoid weight put on and advance weight reduction.

Ingredients:

4 egg whites

2 entire eggs

4 tbsp water

Salt, to taste

Crisply ground dark pepper, to taste

3 tbsp leeks, cleaved

1/2 tsp garlic, minced

Cold squeezed additional virgin olive oil

Directions:

Beat eggs, water, salt, and dark pepper together in a little bowl.

Oil a non-leave skillet with a paper towel plunged in extra-virgin olive oil. Include leeks and garlic, and cook for around 3 to 5 minutes or until delicate. Add cooked leeks and garlic to egg blend.

Empty blend again into oiled griddle and cook until done.

Move omelet onto a plate and embellishment as wanted.

ORIGINAL BIRCHER MUESLI

Muesli was created as a wellbeing nourishment by the Swiss Physician Maximilian Bircher-Brenner towards the finish of the nineteenth century. This is the first muesli formula Mr

Bircher-Benner prescribed to his patients.

Ingredients:

 1 tbsp moved oats

3 tbsp water

1 tbsp improved dense milk

2 tsp lemon juice

1-2 apples (counting skin)

1 tbsp hazelnuts or almonds, ground

Directions:

Join oats and water and refrigerate medium-term. Splashing improves the dietary benefit of oats as it enables catalysts to separate and kill phytic corrosive, an exacerbate that can obstruct the ingestion of numerous minerals in the digestion tracts.

Mesh apples. Include them, together with improved dense milk and lemon juice, to drenched oats. Mix well.

Sprinkle with almonds or hazelnuts and serve.

Did you know?

Drenching improves the dietary benefit of oats as it enables chemicals to separate and kill phytic corrosive, an aggravate that can obstruct the assimilation of numerous minerals in the digestive organs.

FANTASTIC FIBER MUFFINS

Searching for a high-fiber biscuit formula? These morning meal biscuits join wheat grain with entire wheat flour and apples to make a heavenly treat that encourages you arrive at your fiber portion. To sweeten the deal even further, these delectable biscuits are low in fat.

Ingredients:

1/2 cups wheat grain

1 cup nonfat milk (or milk substitute)

1/2 cup unsweetened fruit purée

1 egg

2/3 cup dark colored sugar

1/2 cup generally useful flour

1/2 cup entire wheat flour

1 tsp preparing powder

1 tsp preparing pop

1/2 tsp salt

1 cup natural apples, washed, cored, cleaved

Directions:

Preheat broiler to 375°F (190°C, gas mark 5).

Join wheat grain and drain, and let represent 15 minutes.

In a huge bowl, whisk together fruit purée, egg, and darker

sugar. Mix in wheat blend and blend well.

In a little bowl, consolidate universally handy flour, entire wheat flour, heating powder, preparing pop, and salt. Mix into wheat blend and blend until simply mixed (don't over-blend). Crease in hacked apples.

Fill arranged biscuit cups with hitter (around 66% full). Prepare for around 15-20 minutes.

SALAD

TOMATO, CUCUMBER AND RED ONION SALAD

Low in calories and fat, this serving of mixed greens makes

an extraordinary weight reduction help. In addition, this weight reduction advancing serving of mixed greens contains a lot of onions, a standout amongst other dietary wellsprings of chromium. Chromium has been appeared to help increment or keep up slender weight and help in fat misfortune when joined with work out. These impacts of chromium on body structure are accepted to result from the capacity of this significant follow mineral to upgrade insulin's movement and to improve insulin affectability in the body. The fat misfortune advancing impacts of this serving of mixed greens are additionally reinforced by balsamic vinegar, which not just adds an animating sharpness to this plate of mixed greens however which likewise contains exacerbates that have been appeared to improve the sentiment of satiety and along these lines decrease the measure of nourishment expended.

Ingredients:

2 huge cucumbers, stripped and coarsely hacked

3 huge tomatoes, coarsely hacked

2/3 cup red onion, coarsely hacked

1/3 cup balsamic vinegar

1/2 tbsp white sugar

3 tablespoons additional virgin olive oil

Salt and pepper, to taste

New basil or mint leaves, for embellish (discretionary)

In a huge bowl with a top, join all fixings. Spread, and shake to blend.

Season with salt and pepper.

CHICKEN AND APPLE SALAD

This weight reduction serving of mixed greens formula sets substantial chicken with mouth-watering grapes and crunchy apples to make a taste impression that makes certain to satisfy everybody. Be that as it may, the advantages of this serving of mixed greens are not constrained to culinary sensations; it can likewise be an extraordinary weight reduction help. Chicken conveys a lot of great protein yet is low in starches, while apples contain gelatin, a kind of dietary fiber that restricts the measure of fat our cells assimilate. Gelatin is likewise known to make you feel more full and for a more drawn out time, so you will eat less during the day.

Ingredients:

3 cups cooked chicken, diced

1 cup grapes, divided

1/2 cup celery, diced

3 tbsp red onion, finely slashed

1/2 cup natural apples, diced

6 tbsp additional light mayonnaise

2 tsp lemon juice

Salt and pepper, to taste

Lettuce leaves

Directions:

Join initial five fixings in an enormous bowl.

In a little bowl, join mayonnaise, lemon squeeze, and salt and pepper. Mix into chicken blend.

Organize lettuce leaves on serving plates and top with chicken serving of mixed greens.

SUPER-NUTRITIOUS BROCCOLI SALAD WITH APPLES AND CRANBERRIES

This low-calorie, low-fat plate of mixed greens is made of fixings that are pack brimming with weight reduction supplements, for example, B complex nutrients, calcium, zinc, and iodine. It additionally contains a large number of cell reinforcement supplements, including nutrient C, beta-carotene, quercetin, nutrient E, and selenium, which advance by and large wellbeing.

Ingredients:

4 cups new broccoli florets

1/2 cup dried cranberries

1/2 cup sunflower seeds

3 natural apples

1/4 cup red onion, cleaved

1 cup plain, low-fat yogurt with probiotic microscopic organisms

2 Tbsp Dijon style mustard

1/4 cup nectar

Directions:

Consolidate broccoli florets, dried cranberries, sunflower seeds, cleaved apples, and hacked onion in a huge serving bowl. Mix yogurt, mustard, and nectar in a little bowl.

Add dressing to the plate of mixed greens and hurl. Chill before serving.

GINGER AND CUCUMBER SALAD

Ginger root, a key fixing in this plate of mixed greens, is a fantastic weight reduction help and is in reality found in many weight reduction supplements. Ginger root has craving smothering characteristics, and it has been appeared to fire up the digestion. In one creature study, ginger expanded digestion 20 percent. Moreover, some proof recommends that ginger may likewise be powerful at improving insulin affectability. Likewise cucumber is a magnificent weight reduction nourishment as it contains zero fat and is low in calories.

Ingredients:

2 cucumbers, diced

2 tbsp rice wine vinegar

1 tsp agave nectar

1 tbsp canola oil

1/3 cup salted ginger, depleted

Cleaved mint leaves, to taste

Salt to taste

Directions:

In a medium bowl, join diced cucumbers and ginger.

Whisk together vinegar, agave nectar, canola oil, and mint leaves. Pour over cucumbers and ginger. Hurl and season with salt.

Let marinate refrigerated for 3 hours. Gap onto plates, and trimming as wanted.

ROMAINE AND SMOKED SALMON SALAD

Lettuce is a low calorie vegetable that can be utilized as a reason for weight reduction advancing plates of mixed greens. Be that as it may, it doesn't generally need to be ice shelf lettuce! This simple formula, for instance, utilizes romaine lettuce as a reason for a serving of mixed greens that is brimming with supplements that shed off additional pounds. Romaine lettuce, otherwise called Cos, is stacked with nutrient C, folate, beta-carotene, nutrient K, and manganese. It is likewise a standout amongst other dietary wellsprings of chromium which can assist support with weighting misfortune endeavors. Additionally the crude carrots, radishes, and cucumber in this plate of mixed greens help in weight reduction as they are low in calories while being high in fiber and water. The salmon includes significant protein.

Ingredients:

1 little head natural romaine lettuce

5 ounces smoked salmon, daintily cut

2 tomatoes, diced

4 radishes, daintily cut

1 natural carrot, corner to corner cut

1/2 cucumber, stripped and diced
Juice of a large portion of a lemon

1 tsp new ginger root, stripped and minced

1 tbsp canola oil

Directions:

Orchestrate romaine lettuce on two plates. Top with salmon, tomatoes, radishes, carrots, and cucumber.

Shake lemon juice, canola oil, and minced ginger in firmly

secured container. Pour over plate of mixed greens.

CARROT FENNEL CUCUMBER SALAD

This summery serving of mixed greens works like enchantment to calm your spirit—and to consume abundance fat. While being amazingly low in calories, this plate of mixed greens is pressed with fiber and nutrient C. It likewise contains some fundamental unsaturated fats.

Ingredients:

6 natural carrots, meagerly cut

1 fennel bulb, meagerly cut

1 cucumber, meagerly cut

1 cup crisp parsley, slashed

4 tbsp naturally crushed lemon juice

2 tbsp additional virgin olive oil

Ocean salt

Newly ground dark pepper

Directions:

Consolidate carrots, fennel, cucumber, and parsley in an enormous bowl.

Blend lemon juice, olive oil, salt, and pepper in a compartment with a securable top. Fix cover and shake.

Pour dressing over plate of mixed greens and hurl delicately.

BEET AND CARROT SALAD WITH GINGER

This formula sets beets with carrots to make a profoundly nutritious serving of mixed greens that is stuffed with fiber and nutrients while being low in calories.

Ingredients:

1/2 cup crude beets, stripped and ground

1/2 cup natural carrots, ground

2 tbsp squeezed apple

1 tbsp extra-virgin olive oil

1/2 tsp new ginger, minced

1/8 tsp ocean salt

Directions:

Consolidate ground beets and carrots in a little bowl.

Blend squeezed apple, olive oil, ginger, and salt in a different astonish and sprinkle plate of mixed greens blend. Hurl tenderly. Appreciate!

Did you know?

Beta-carotene, found in numerous orange vegetables, for example, carrots, is a fat-soluble nutrient, which implies that it must be expended together with a tad of fat with the end goal for it to be retained and used by the body. Along these lines, the basic unsaturated fats gave by the olive oil in this formula are a perfect backup for carrots.

SOUP

APPLE AND ONION SOUP

An apple daily repels the specialist, goes the familiar saying. Be that as it may, did you realize that apples can likewise fend off overabundance pounds? Apples contain gelatin, a kind of dietary fiber that constrains the measure of fat our cells ingest. Additionally onions help keep

abundance pounds under
control: onions are outstanding
amongst other dietary wellsprings
of chromium, a mineral that can
help increment or keep up fit
weight and help in fat misfortune
when joined with work out.

Ingredients:

1 Tbsp canola oil

2 medium yellow onions, cut

1 little leek, cleaved

1/2 Tbsp new rosemary, slashed

1/2 Tbsp new thyme

3 natural apples, cut into little
dices

6 cups without fat, low-sodium vegetable juices

Directions:

Warmth the oil in a medium pot over medium warmth. Include the onions and sauté until brilliant.

Pour in the stock and bring to the bubble over medium-high warmth. Include the apples, and decrease the warmth to medium-low.

Stew for 10 minutes.

HOT TOMATO SOUP

This soup is plentiful in chromium, a mineral that may help increment or keep up fit weight and help in fat misfortune when joined with work out. These impacts of chromium on body sythesis are accepted to result from the capacity of this significant follow mineral to upgrade insulin's action and to improve insulin affectability in the body. In addition, the bean stew and garlic highlighted in this weight reduction soup are wealthy in phytochemicals that expansion the rate at which your body consumes vitality.

Ingredients:

3 huge garlic cloves

3 oz shallots, stripped cut

1 tablespoon olive oil

1 (14 1/2-ounce) can stewed tomatoes, undrained

1/2 cups chicken juices

1/2 teaspoon bean stew powder

1/2 tsp apple juice vinegar

1/4 tsp salt

Run of naturally ground red pepper

2 tbsp crisp basil, slashed

Directions:

Strip and squash garlic and put in a safe spot. Leaving squashed or minced garlic for at any rate 5-10 minutes in the wake of smashing expands its wellbeing defensive impacts.

While wellbeing advancing mixes are framing in squashed garlic, consolidate shallots, tomatoes, chicken stock, and apple juice vinegar in a blender or nourishment processor and procedure until smooth.

Warmth olive oil in an enormous nonstick pan over medium warmth. Include garlic and bean stew powder, and cook around 30 seconds, mixing continually.

Include tomato blend, and heat to the point of boiling. Mood killer warmth and mix in basil. Serve hot.

WHOLESOME WINTER PEA AND WATERCRESS SOUP (DAIRY-FREE)

This weight reduction soup with a compelling smooth surface is extremely low in calories; yet, it conveys an astounding measure of nutrient C. Research has demonstrated an immediate connection between low blood levels of nutrient C and expanded fat gathering, especially around the abdomen. Besides, on account of the watercress, this soup is pressed with calcium which has been appeared to advance weight reduction. Watercress is additionally low in oxalic corrosive, an intensify that can repress the assimilation of calcium from numerous different plants nourishments.

Ingredients:

1 huge onion

1 garlic clove

6 cups vegetable or chicken stock

1 zucchini

30 oz solidified peas

3 oz watercress

Salt and pepper, to taste

Directions:

Strip and smash the garlic and put in a safe spot. Leaving

squashed or minced garlic for in any event 5-10 minutes subsequent to pounding augments its wellbeing defensive impacts.

While wellbeing advancing mixes are shaping in squashed garlic, wash and trim the zucchini, and cut it into pieces.

Strip and slash the onion, and sweat it, together with the minced garlic, in 2-3 tablespoons of chicken or vegetable stock in a stock pot.

Include the zucchini pieces and pour in the remainder of the stock. Heat to the point of boiling and stew for until the zucchini lumps are simply cooked, around 10 minutes.

Include the solidified peas and stew for 3 minutes. Include the watercress and stew for one more moment.

Expel from the warmth and let cool for a couple of moments. Procedure with a hand-held blender until smooth. Season with salt.

LENTIL CHILI SOUP

This hot soup can assist you with consuming fat as it is wealthy in capsaicin, the fixing that gives bean stew its sharp flavor. Capsaicin is celebrated for its capacity to expand the rate at which the body consumes vitality, making it a phenomenal weight reduction help. Besides, this soup is wealthy in protein and

fiber which help keep your
glucose levels on a level.

Ingredients:

2 tbsp additional virgin olive oil

1 enormous yellow onion, cut

2 carrots, diced

2 cloves garlic

1/2 tsp bean stew powder

1 tsp cumin

1 tsp dried oregano

1 cup red lentils

28 oz (420g) canned tomatoes

6 cups vegetable stock

1/2 tsp salt

1/2 tsp dark pepper, crisply
ground

Directions:

Strip and pound garlic and put in
a safe spot. Leaving squashed or
minced garlic for in any event 5-
10 minutes in the wake of
pulverizing will amplify its
wellbeing advancing impacts.

While wellbeing advancing mixes
are shaping in squashed garlic,
heat olive oil in an enormous
nonstick pan over medium
warmth. Include onion and cook
for 3 minutes, mixing at times.

Include stock, lentils, carrots,
bean stew powder, cumin,
oregano, salt, and pepper, and
bring to bubble. Spread pot and

let stew for 25 minutes over medium warmth.

Include garlic and let stew for an additional 5 minutes.

Spoon soup into people bowls and serve hot.

NOURISHING NETTLE SOUP

Amazingly low in calories and high in nutrients and minerals, bother is an incredible plant for anybody resolved to lose fat. Know, in any case, that bother has solid diuretic properties, and in this manner a portion of the lost pounds will in actuality be water. Likewise yogurt—which is utilized to decorate this captivating, jade green soup— helps support the muscle to fat ratio's consuming forces and advance weight reduction.

Ingredients:

6 oz youthful annoy tips

4 oz new spinach

2 tbsp olive oil

2 shallots, hacked

2 cups water

2 cups skimmed natural milk

3 tbsp flour

Run of ground white pepper

Run of ground nutmeg

Salt to taste

Yogurt with probiotic microscopic organisms, for decorate

Directions:

Wash annoy and spinach completely. Deplete and slash coarsely.

Warmth olive oil and sauté onion in an enormous pan until brilliant darker.

Include water, annoy, and spinach, and heat to the point of boiling. Cook until annoy and spinach are delicate. Mix with a hand held blender until smooth.

Whisk cold drain and flour together in a little bowl. Fill pot and speed to mix completely.

Heat to the point of boiling and stew for a couple of moments, until thickened. Season with salt, white pepper, and nutmeg. Expel from heat.

Empty soup into serving bowls and enhancement with a whirl of yogurt. Serve.

Note: As weeds are wealthy in nitrates, they ought not be devoured by small kids, individuals with gout, or others with a condition that requires a low-nitrate diet.

Did you know?

Nitrates, inorganic exacerbates that can mess wellbeing up in the event that they transform into nitrites in the body, gather normally in numerous plants including bramble and spinach. In any case, you can limit the nitrate substance of your bother dishes by just devouring youthful annoy shoots and by maintaining a strategic distance from manure zones and toilets when picking brambles. You can likewise decrease the chances of nitrates transforming into nitrites by devouring a savor rich nutrient C or potentially E alongside your bother dish — these nutrients are exceptionally viable at averting the transformation of nitrates into nitrites.

BARLEY SOUP WITH CARROTS AND PARSLEY

Grain is a hero grain for any individual who needs to get in shape. In addition to the fact that barley is low in calories, it additionally has the most reduced Glycemic Index (GI) rating of every normal grain. Low glycemic nourishments help keep the degrees of fat-putting away hormones low and diminish sugar yearnings. Additionally the low-calorie yogurt and the fiber-rich carrots in this soup add to the fat-consuming ability of this sound soup.

Ingredients:

2/3 cup water

1/3 cup pearled grain

2 tbsp additional virgin olive oil

1/2 cup yellow onion, slashed

1 cup carrots

2 cups vegetable stock

1 2/3 cup plain yogurt containing probiotic microorganisms

2/3 cup crisp parsley, minced

Salt and pepper, to taste

1/2 tsp dark pepper, naturally ground.

Directions:

Heat water to the point of boiling in a soup pot. Include grain and let stew secured for around 25-30 minutes over low warmth. When water has vanished, expel from warmth and put in a safe spot

In a stock pot, cook onion in olive oil over medium warmth for 4-5 minutes until delicate. Include stock and carrots and bring to bubble. Diminish to a stew, spread, and cook for 20 minutes.

Include cooked grain and let stew one more moment or two. Expel from heat.

Mix in yogurt and seasonings. Serve right away.

CHICKEN SOUP WITH RICE AND GREEN PEAS

Chicken and green peas sneak up all of a sudden however have an exceptionally low glycemic list rating, making this appetizing soup perfect for anybody attempting to shed off additional pounds. Chicken is additionally a decent wellspring of B nutrients, for example, nutrient B3 and nutrient B6, which are significant for fruitful weight reduction.

Ingredients:

4 cups sans fat, low-sodium chicken juices

1 little onion, slashed

1/2 cups green peas

2 little ribs natural celery, diced

2 little carrots, cut

1/2 cup short grain darker rice, washed

2 cups skinless, natural chicken, cooked and diced

Directions:

Absorb rice cold water from 15 minutes to 60 minutes. This will diminish cooking time.

Heat soup to the point of boiling in an enormous pot. Include presoaked rice and vegetables. Diminish warmth to low, cover and stew, blending incidentally, until rice is delicate.

Include cooked chicken and stew for 3-4 minutes.

Did you know?

Together with customarily developed ringer peppers, traditionally developed celery is up there at the highest priority on the rundown of vegetables that contain the most elevated levels of contaminants, including neurotoxic pesticides and chlorothalonil (a potential cancer-causing agent)). That is the reason it is profoundly fitting to settle on naturally developed produce when purchasing celery.

CHICKEN AND BARLEY SOUP

Grain is an incredible grain for anybody needing to shed off overabundance pounds. It is low in calories and has the most minimal Glycemic Index (GI) rating of every single regular grain. The protein-rich chicken in this soup further brings down the glycemic heap of this phenomenal weight reduction supper.

Ingredients:

1/2 pounds skinless chicken bosom

9 cups chicken juices

1 cup carrots, diced

1/2 cup natural celery, finely slashed

1/2 cup grain, cooked [buy natural grain here]

1/4 cup yellow onion, cut

1/2 cup crisp spinach leaves, cut into strips

Salt and pepper, to taste.

Directions:

Cut the chicken bosoms into reduced down pieces. Spot in a

huge stockpot and spread with juices.

Heat to the point of boiling and skim surface of aggregated froth. Stew on low warmth for around 40 minutes.

Include carrots, celery, and onion and stew for an additional 15 minutes.

Include spinach and grain. Warmth through and season with salt and pepper.

THE
END…………………………………
…

Made in the USA
Monee, IL
06 December 2020